ANXIETY RELIEF GUIDE FOR DOGS

Holistic Healing Approach with Homeopathy

Dr Baron Harper Sagewood

DISCLAIMER

This book is intended to provide general information and knowledge of Anxiety Relief for Dogs using Homeopathy. It is not intended to be a substitute for professional medical or mental health advice, diagnosis, or treatment. The information provided in this book is based on my personal experiences and research, and may not be applicable or relevant to every individual's unique situation. I am not responsible for any errors or omissions, and make no guarantees or warranties regarding the accuracy, completeness, or suitability of the information provided. Readers should consult with a qualified medical or mental health professional before making any decisions about their health or well-being based on the information provided in this book. I disclaim any liability for any damages or injuries arising from the use or total reliance on the information provided in this book.

DEDICATION

To all the devoted dog owners and their beloved furry companions,

This book is dedicated to you, the compassionate souls who strive to understand and alleviate the anxiety that our canine friends may face. Your unwavering love, patience, and commitment to providing a safe and comforting environment for your dogs inspire us deeply.

May this book serve as a guiding light, offering valuable insights and effective solutions to bring peace and serenity to your furry companions' lives. Your devotion to their well-being is a testament to the beautiful bond between humans and dogs.

In honor of the countless tail wags, affectionate licks, and moments of unconditional love, we dedicate "Anxiety Relief for Dogs" to you. May your journey together be filled with joy, understanding, and a lifetime of cherished memories.

Table of Contents

INTRODUCTION

Welcome to Anxiety Relief Guide for Dogs: A Holistic Healing Approach with Homeopathy. This comprehensive guide is your passport to the world of natural solutions, designed to embrace and support your cherished canine companion through times of anxiety. As an experienced Veterinary Doctor, I am elated to share my expertise, unveiling the wonders of homeopathy in managing and alleviating anxiety in dogs.

Within these pages, we shall embark on a fascinating journey into the realm of homeopathy—a healing art with deep roots in history, spanning centuries. At its heart lies the profound concept of "like cures like," harnessing the power of highly diluted natural substances to ignite the body's innate healing capabilities. In contrast to the mere suppression of symptoms, homeopathy targets the root causes, rendering a gentle and non-invasive path to tranquility.

Chapter 1 sets the stage, unveiling the enigmatic aspects of canine anxiety. By discerning the signs, triggers, and repercussions of anxiety, you will become a steadfast guardian, equipped with the knowledge to provide your four-legged friend with the best care imaginable. Understanding the core reasons behind their unease empowers you to craft a bespoke homeopathic treatment plan tailored to your furry companion's individual needs.

The second chapter invites you to traverse time, delving into the origins and timeless principles of homeopathy. This insightful voyage will foster a deep appreciation for this ancient healing wisdom and its evolutionary journey. Central to homeopathy is the art of personalized treatment, cherishing the uniqueness of each canine soul, making it an artful approach to managing anxiety.

Venturing further, we embark on the heart of our odyssey, exploring a treasure trove of homeopathic remedies crafted to soothe canine anxiety. With intricate discussions on the properties and indications of each remedy, you will be empowered to make well-informed choices for your beloved companion's well-being.

As a Veterinary Doctor, I understand the potency of blending diverse healing modalities. In Chapter 4, we uncover the seamless integration of homeopathy with traditional veterinary care, forging a comprehensive path to anxiety relief in dogs.

Chapter 5 shines a light on the diverse manifestations of anxiety in dogs, arising from an array of triggers such as thunderstorms, fireworks, and separation anxiety. Armed with this knowledge, you will explore the realm of homeopathic solutions, becoming a beacon of comfort for your precious pet.

While homeopathy plays a pivotal role in anxiety management, Chapter 6 unveils the art of behavioral training, synergistically united with homeopathy to foster emotional resilience and overall well-being in your furry friend.

Throughout this book, real-life case studies grace Chapter 7, narrating inspiring anecdotes of anxiety relief in dogs through the magic of homeopathy. These heartwarming tales illuminate the practical applications of homeopathic remedies, their transformative impact on canine behavior, and the blossoming of serene companionship.

In Chapter 8, we humbly glean wisdom from esteemed veterinary homeopaths, passionate pioneers dedicated to this cherished field. Their insights elevate our understanding of homeopathic anxiety relief for dogs, expanding the tapestry of knowledge.

Chapter 9 highlights the role of nutrition in the holistic tapestry of canine well-being.

Discover how specific dietary tweaks and supplements can bolster and complement the homeopathic treatment, nurturing serenity within your anxious pet.

Mindfulness and relaxation techniques, the essence of Chapter 10, bring peace to the forefront. Infuse these practices into your dog's daily routine, harmonizing their inner world and empowering them to master stress and anxiety.

Chapter 11 unveils the art of crafting a tranquil haven for your canine companion. Forge a sanctuary, enveloped in calming energies, where your dog can feel secure and embrace moments of respite.

The medicinal prowess of herbs takes center stage in Chapter 12, illuminating nature's gentle balm for canine anxiety, another facet of holistic healing.

Chapter 13 is dedicated to the challenge of separation anxiety, a hurdle faced by many dog owners. Herein lies a guide to assuage this heartache and navigate the storm of emotions.

Chapter 14 beckons us to decode the subtle language of our canine friends, tapping into the beauty of their signals and emotions, fortifying the bonds of our timeless friendship.

Finally, our journey concludes in Chapter 15, with a glimpse into the future of homeopathic anxiety relief for dogs. Witness the ever-evolving frontier of this captivating field, where innovation paves the way for brighter tomorrows.

Throughout this enlightening quest, I shall be your trusted companion, illuminating your path with profound explanations, answering your queries, and guiding you toward mastering the art of homeopathic anxiety relief for dogs. Together, we shall nurture an oasis of comfort and tranquility for our cherished furry companions. Let this odyssey commence, and may the gentle embrace of homeopathy be your beacon of solace.

CHAPTER 1: CRACKING THE CODE OF CANINE ANXIETY

Anxiety—it's not just a human thing. Our adorable pups experience it too! But fear not, understanding their emotions doesn't require a secret language decoder. In this thrilling chapter, we're off on a quest to uncover the mysteries of doggie anxiety—the telltale signs, the triggers that spark it, and how it affects our furry buddies.

1.1 Signs And Symptoms: The Unmistakable Clues

Our canine pals might not talk like we do, but they have their unique ways of expressing emotions. Look out for these little hints or big declarations of anxiety:

1. *Barking Bonanza:* When anxiety hits, barking becomes their megaphone—especially when they encounter strange things or loud noises.

2. *Battle of the Growls:* Fear can turn them into little warriors, growling to protect themselves from what they see as threats.

3. Wrecking Havoc: A lonely pooch might turn into a mini bulldozer, chewing, digging, or tearing stuff up to let off steam.

4. Trembling Tales: Their bodies might quiver like jelly, showing off the jitters of anxiety.

5. Gasping for Comfort: An anxious pup may pant like a marathon runner, even when they're not running at all.

6. Seeking Solitude: When feeling overwhelmed, they might retreat to a quiet spot to find some peace.

7. A Slump in the Stomach: Stress can lead to a loss of appetite or strange eating habits.

8. Lick Attack: An anxious pooch might lick itself constantly, trying to calm its nerves.

1.2 Unraveling The Triggers: What Sends Their Hearts Racing

Every puzzle has its pieces, and anxiety has its triggers. Discover the common culprits that stir up canine anxiety:

1. Clamor and Chaos: Thunderstorms, fireworks, or noisy construction work can rattle their nerves.

2. The Dreaded Alone Time: Being left alone for too long can be super stressful and trigger separation anxiety.

3. Change and Uncertainty: Moving to a new home or big changes in the family can make them feel uneasy.

4. The Need for Friends: Early life without enough socialization can lead to anxiety about meeting new buddies.

5. Scars of the Past: Past traumas can cast a long shadow, causing anxiety to rear its head.

6. Health Matters: Being sick or in pain can make anxiety even worse.

1.3 The Impact On Their Happy Tails: How Anxiety Affects Them

Anxiety isn't just a passing storm—it can cast a cloud over their lives, affecting them in many ways:

1. *Immune System Shake-Up:* Anxiety weakens their defense, making them more prone to illnesses.

2. *Tummy Turmoil:* Stress can upset the tummy, leading to digestion issues and wonky eating habits.

3. *Adding to the Struggle:* If they already have health problems, anxiety can make things even tougher for them.

4. *A Behavior Balancing Act:* Anxiety can mess with their behavior, making them act out or become withdrawn.

5. *The Quest for Joy:* Anxiety can dampen their happy moments, leaving them feeling less joyful.

CHAPTER 2: UNVEILING THE MAGIC OF HOMEOPATHY: A JOURNEY BACK IN TIME

Homeopathy, a remarkable healing system that has stood the test of over two centuries, is more than just medicine—it's a holistic approach to restoring harmony in the body. In this captivating chapter, we'll dive into the roots of homeopathy, explore its core principles, and see how it works wonders in relieving anxiety in our adorable canine pals.

2.1 The Birth Of Homeopathy

A bold German physician named Samuel Hahnemann, dissatisfied with the medical practices of his time, embarks on a daring experiment. He tests various substances on himself and volunteers, observing how they trigger symptoms similar to the very illnesses they were meant to cure. And so, the seeds of homeopathy were sown.

Hahnemann cleverly coined the term "homeopathy," blending "homoios" (similar) and "pathos" (suffering) from Greek, to capture the essence of "like cures like." The core idea? A substance that can cause symptoms in a healthy person can also heal someone with similar symptoms.

2.2 Unraveling The Homeopathic Marvels

Homeopathy's enchanting ways are guided by some fascinating principles:

1 The Law of Similars

Picture this again: like a gentle puzzle solver, homeopathy treats the "Law of Similars" as its guide. If a substance can create certain symptoms in a healthy soul, it can charm those same symptoms away in someone unwell. It's all about finding that perfect match!

2 A Dance of Individuality

In the magical world of homeopathy, no two beings are alike. Each patient is treated as an exceptional individual. It's not just about the disease—it's about their whole being! Homeopaths keenly observe their physical, emotional, and mental aspects, crafting a unique remedy just for them.

3 The Secret of the Tiny Dose

In this sorcery, less is more! Homeopathic remedies undergo a mystical process called "potentization." Through delicate dilution and vigorous shaking, the remedy's energy is unleashed while minimizing any toxic effects. It's all about preserving the essence of healing magic.

4 The Dance of Potency

Enter the realm of "potency," a scale represented by "X" or "C." The higher the potency, the greater the dilution, and the stronger the magic! These powerful spells retain their healing prowess while bidding farewell to harmful side effects.

2.3 Homeopathy And Our Furry Friends

Now, let's see how homeopathy works wonders in soothing the souls of our beloved canine companions. Picture this again: a dog quaking with fear during a thunderstorm, restless and trembling. Homeopathy steps in like a guardian angel, offering a remedy that mirrors those exact symptoms in a healthy person.

Homeopathic remedies for canine anxiety come in liquid, tablet, or pellet forms—convenient magic for our furry friends! The key to unlocking the perfect remedy lies in observing their unique symptoms and seeking the guidance of a wise veterinary homeopath.

CHAPTER 3: MAGIC POTIONS FOR CALM CANINES

In this enchanting chapter, we'll explore a collection of homeopathic wonders—potions that whisk away anxiety from our canine companions. Homeopathy's treasure trove is brimming with remedies crafted from nature's gifts, each with its special power. To work this magic, we must discover the ideal remedy, tailored to their symptoms and quirks. Are you ready to join this mystical adventure? Let's begin!

3.1 Aconitum Napellus (Aconite)

Behold Aconitum, the brave one! It's a remedy for sudden, intense anxiety triggered by wild storms or traumatic events. A dog trembling with fear, desperately seeking an escape from the chaos—Aconitum comes to the rescue. Administered at the first sign of anxiety, it works its magic swiftly.

3.2 Arsenicum Album
(Arsenicum)

Say hello to Arsenicum, the comforter! This remedy soothes dogs facing anxiety from separation or changes in their environment. A restless pup seeking reassurance and plagued by tummy troubles—Arsenicum waves its wand, bringing relief. Perfect for those long hours alone!

3.3 Gelsemium Sempervirens
(Gelsemium)

Meet Gelsemium, the anticipator! When a dog frets over upcoming events, like vet visits or car rides, Gelsemium is the remedy to call upon. Trembling legs, weakness, and a desire to hide away—all fade away under Gelsemium's enchantment.

3.4 Phosphorus

Here's Phosphorus, the empathetic friend! When a dog feels deeply connected to their human emotions, Phosphorus is their savior. Seeking constant affection and anxiety in the dark or during thunderstorms—Phosphorus waves its wand, easing their woes.

3.5 Pulsatilla Nigricans (Pulsatilla)

Enter Pulsatilla, the emotionally dependent one! For dogs easily distressed by changes and seeking comfort, Pulsatilla is the remedy to turn to. A clingy companion anxious when separated from their human—Pulsatilla's enchantment brings a sense of calm.

3.6 Ignatia Amara (Ignatia)

Behold Ignatia, the healer of hearts! When a dog faces anxiety and grief due to loss, Ignatia's magic mends its broken spirits. Sudden mood swings, inconsolable sadness—Ignatia's spell works wonders, soothing their aching souls.

CHAPTER 4: HOMEOPATHY AND TRADITIONAL VETERINARY CARE

In this chapter, we will study the advantages of mixing homeopathy with standard veterinarian therapy for anxiety alleviation in dogs. Both homeopathy and conventional veterinary medication have their strengths, and when used together, they may offer a potent and well-rounded approach to resolving canine anxiety. By integrating the holistic principles of homeopathy with evidence-based veterinary therapies, we can offer complete care for our beloved animal friends.

4.1 Complementing Treatment Modalities

Homeopathy and regular veterinarian therapy are not mutually incompatible; rather, they may complement one another to produce the best possible results for dogs with anxiety. While traditional therapies may concentrate on controlling physical symptoms or underlying medical disorders, homeopathy addresses the emotional and energetic components of the dog's well-being.

For instance, if a dog is suffering anxiety due to a medical condition, such as chronic pain or an infection, typical veterinarian care may entail drugs and particular therapies to address the physical discomfort. At the same time, homeopathy may play a significant role in supporting the dog's emotional condition, lowering stress, and boosting general recovery.

4.2 Reducing The Use Of Pharmaceuticals

One of the great benefits of combining homeopathy with regular veterinary treatment is the ability to lessen the dependency on pharmaceutical medicines, particularly for long-term anxiety control. While pharmaceuticals might be required in some cases, they may come with possible side effects or hazards.

Homeopathic treatments, being natural and mild, may be used with or instead of medications in certain instances. They provide a safe option for controlling anxiety, particularly for dogs with allergies or contraindications to specific medicines.

4.3 Enhancing Overall Well-being

The combination of homeopathy and standard veterinarian treatment may boost the dog's general well-being. Homeopathic treatments are noted for their holistic approach, treating the complete being of the dog rather than simply the apparent symptoms. By evaluating the dog's emotional, mental, and physical health, we may encourage a deeper degree of healing and harmony.

For example, if a dog is suffering anxiety due to a particular medical procedure, such as surgery, a well-structured treatment plan may combine pain management with conventional pharmaceuticals, coupled with homeopathic treatments to minimize pre and post-operative tension and anxiety.

4.4 Individualized Treatment Plans

Integrating homeopathy with regular veterinary care allows for the creation of personalized treatment strategies suited to each dog's particular requirements. Homeopathy's focus on individualization meshes wonderfully with the notion of tailored veterinary treatment.

By evaluating the dog's temperament, history, environmental circumstances, and individual anxiety triggers, we may build a tailored strategy that takes into consideration both conventional and homeopathic therapies. This combination enhances the probability of a good result and a happier, less stressed canine partner.

4.5 Collaboration Between Professionals

To guarantee a successful combination of homeopathic and standard veterinary treatment, communication between specialists is necessary. Veterinarians and licensed veterinary homeopaths may work together, exchanging information and ideas to build a coherent treatment plan.

Open communication provides for a thorough awareness of the dog's entire health and well-being, leading to educated judgments on the most suitable therapies.

CHAPTER 5: ADDRESSING SPECIFIC ANXIETY TRIGGERS IN DOGS

In this chapter, we will investigate particular anxiety triggers typically experienced by dogs and how homeopathy, coupled with behavioral approaches, may be used to manage them successfully. Understanding and managing these triggers are vital in providing holistic care for our canine friends, helping them navigate through anxiety-inducing circumstances with confidence and ease.

5.1 Thunderstorm Phobia

Thunderstorms may be a substantial cause of worry for many pets. The loud booms, blinding flashes of lightning, and changes in air pressure may induce panic and stress reactions. To combat thunderstorm anxiety in dogs, we might explore the following approaches:

- *Homeopathic Remedies:* Aconitum napellus is commonly used for dogs suffering extreme anxiety during thunderstorms. Gelsemium sempervirens may also be good for anticipatory anxiety before a storm.

Additionally, Phosphorus may be good for dogs who are sensitive to atmospheric changes.

- *Safe spot:* Create a designated safe spot in your house where your dog may take sanctuary during storms. This place should be pleasant and familiar, with access to their favorite toys and bedding.

- *Calming methods:* Calming methods such as gentle massage, TTouch (Tellington Touch), and giving comfortable white noise may help distract and relax frightened dogs during thunderstorms.

5.2 Fireworks Anxiety

Fireworks displays may be unpleasant for dogs owing to the loud sounds and dazzling lighting. To decrease fireworks fear, we might consider the following strategies:

- *Homeopathic Remedies:* Similar to thunderstorm phobia, Aconitum napellus, and Gelsemium sempervirens may be beneficial for acute anxiety during fireworks displays.

- *Desensitization:* Gradually expose your dog to recorded firework noises at a low level while offering positive reinforcement and treats. Over time, raise the level to gradually desensitize your dog to the sounds.

- *Behavior Modification*: Engage your dog in enjoyable and engaging activities during fireworks displays to distract them from the noise. Provide engaging toys or play games to refocus their concentration.

5.3 Separation Anxiety

Separation anxiety is a typical problem encountered by dogs when they are left alone. To assist dogs deal with separation anxiety, explore the following approaches:

- *Homeopathic Remedies*: Arsenicum album is commonly used for dogs with separation anxiety. Pulsatilla nigricans may also be good for dogs who grow worried while away from their owners.

- *Gradual Departures*: eventually expand the time you are gone from your dog, beginning with brief periods and eventually increasing the duration. This may help them get more acclimated to your absence.

- *Pre-Departure Routine*: Establish a regular pre-departure routine that helps indicate to your dog that you will return. Providing a unique gift or toy upon departing might generate good connections with your departure.

5.4 Veterinary Visits And White Coat Anxiety

Many dogs develop anxiety while visiting the veterinarian owing to new situations and encounters with strangers. To relieve veterinarian visit anxiety, explore the following strategies:

- *Homeopathic Remedies:* Gelsemium sempervirens may be good for anticipatory anxiety before veterinarian consultations. Ignatia Amara may also be good for dogs suffering anxiety and sadness due to vet appointments.

- *Counterconditioning:* Pair good experiences with veterinarian appointments by bringing treats or toys to reward your dog during and after the visit.

- *Familiarization Visits:* Take your dog to the veterinarian clinic for quick, pleasant visits without any medical treatments involved. This might help them get more comfortable with the setting.

CHAPTER 6: BEHAVIORAL TRAINING AND HOMEOPATHY

In this chapter, we will study the synergistic combination of behavioral training and homeopathy in resolving canine anxiety. Behavioral training tries to change undesired habits and teach coping methods, while homeopathy offers gentle and comprehensive assistance for the emotional well-being of dogs. By mixing these two techniques, we may build a strong pair to successfully treat anxiety and foster beneficial behavioral changes in our loving canine friends.

6.1 Understanding Behavioral Training For Anxiety Relief:

Behavioral training combines positive reward and conditioning to improve a dog's behavior to anxiety-inducing events. The idea is to teach dogs alternative behaviors and coping strategies that replace nervous responses with calm and relaxed activities.

1 Desensitization

Desensitization is a frequent behavioral approach used for anxiety alleviation. It includes gradual exposure to the anxiety trigger at a low intensity, combined with positive reinforcement and incentives. Over time, the exposure amount is raised in a regulated way, helping the dog grow more tolerant and less reactive to the trigger.

For example, if a dog is frightened of strangers, desensitization may include progressively exposing the dog to new individuals at a distance where they feel comfortable. As the dog feels more at ease, the distance is lessened, and a positive reward is offered for calm behavior.

2 Counterconditioning

Counterconditioning includes linking anxiety stimuli with good experiences to influence the dog's emotional reaction. This is done by matching the anxiety trigger with something nice or gratifying.

For instance, if a dog is frightened during vehicle journeys, counterconditioning may entail offering the dog food or toys every time they get into the car. Over time, the dog may grow to link automobile journeys with happy events, lowering their fear.

6.2 Integrating Homeopathy With Behavioral Training

Homeopathy may considerably boost the efficacy of behavioral training for anxiety reduction in dogs. By treating the underlying emotional imbalances and energy disturbances, homeopathy may help dogs stay more responsive to behavioral training strategies.

1 Selecting Homeopathic Remedies

When combining homeopathy with behavioral training, the selection of the most suitable remedy is vital. Homeopathic medicines that match the dog's individual emotional and mental symptoms may assist in lowering anxiety and boosting receptivity to training.

For example, if a dog displays anticipatory worry before automobile journeys, Gelsemium sempervirens may be given as a homeopathic treatment to assist reduce their anxiousness, making the training process more successful.

2 Individualized Treatment Plans

Homeopathy's focus on individualization meshes wonderfully with behavioral training's tailored approach. Combining these two methods enables the formulation of individualized treatment regimens based on the dog's unique traits and particular anxiety triggers.

By addressing both the behavioral and emotional elements of the dog, we can build a complete strategy that treats the fundamental cause of the anxiety and encourages sustainable improvements in behavior.

6.3 Patience And Consistency

Both behavioral training and homeopathy need patience and persistence to obtain favorable effects. Training sessions should be performed frequently and in a peaceful, supportive setting. Homeopathic treatments may take time to exhibit their full benefits, therefore continuous administration is crucial.

6.4 Professional Guidance

To guarantee the proper integration of behavioral training and homeopathy, it is important to seek expert supervision. Certified animal behaviorists and veterinary homeopaths may give professional insights and build a coherent treatment plan adapted to the individual requirements of the dog.

CHAPTER 7: CASE STUDIES - SUCCESS STORIES OF ANXIETY RELIEF IN DOGS

In this chapter, we will analyze real-life case studies of dogs that have received anxiety reduction through the combination of behavioral training and homeopathy. These success stories show the usefulness of this strong combination in treating numerous anxiety triggers and fostering mental well-being in our loving canine friends. Each case study highlights the transforming effect of a holistic strategy that incorporates the particular needs and features of the dogs.

Case Study 1: Thunderstorm Phobia

Dog: Max, a 5-year-old Labrador Retriever

Symptoms: Max would get highly worried and agitated during thunderstorms. He would pace, pant excessively, and seek sanctuary beneath furniture or in closets. His anxiousness would rise with each loud clap of thunder, and he would shiver uncontrollably.

Treatment Approach: Max's owner, Sarah, sought the services of a trained veterinary behaviorist and a veterinary homeopath. The behaviorist proposed a desensitization procedure, where they progressively exposed Max to recorded thunderstorm noises at a low intensity, praising him for keeping quiet. The volume was progressively raised over time as Max got more comfortable.

In combination with the desensitization program, a homeopathic medicine, Gelsemium sempervirens, was recommended by the veterinary homeopath. The treatment helped relieve Max's anticipatory worry before the storms and boosted his emotional resilience during thunderstorms.

Results: Over many weeks of continuous training and homeopathic medication, Max's sensitivity to thunderstorms started to alter. He displayed less stress and shaking, and his pacing lessened dramatically. While not cured of his phobia, Max grew visibly more peaceful during storms, seeking comfort from his owner rather than hiding.

Case Study 2: Separation Anxiety

Dog: Bella, a 3-year-old Toy Poodle

Symptoms: Bella would grow agitated anytime her owner, Michael, left the home. She would bark continuously, claw at doors, and urinate in the home when left alone. Bella's separation anxiety was generating major stress for both her and Michael.

Treatment Approach: Michael sought help from a trained veterinary behaviorist and a veterinary homeopath to handle Bella's separation anxiety. The behaviorist proposed a progressive departure pattern, where Michael would leave the home for small intervals and gradually extend the time away, always offering positive reinforcement upon his return.

For Bella's emotional support, the veterinary homeopath administered the homeopathic medication Arsenicum album. This solution tackled Bella's fear of abandonment and gave gentle assistance throughout her training.

Results: With continuous training and homeopathic therapy, Bella's separation anxiety started to reduce. She grew more tolerant of Michael's absences and displayed less disruptive behavior. Over time, Bella's discomfort diminished, and she learned to wait calmly for Michael's return without excessive barking or urinating.

Case Study 3: Fireworks Anxiety

Dog: Rocky, a 4-year-old Boxer

Symptoms: Rocky would get highly agitated and afraid during fireworks shows. He would pant heavily, slobber excessively, and seek to hide in tiny locations, such as closets or under furniture.

Treatment Approach: Rocky's owner, Amanda, hired a trained veterinary behaviorist and a veterinary homeopath to treat his fireworks fear. The behaviorist advocated counterconditioning by connecting the sound of distant fireworks with joyful activities, such as playing or reward puzzles.

To promote Rocky's emotional well-being, the veterinary homeopath ordered a homeopathic medicine, Aconitum napellus, to be taken before the commencement of the fireworks displays. This cure attempted to calm Rocky's extreme anxiousness during the pyrotechnics.

Results: With the combination of counterconditioning and homeopathic therapy, Rocky's reaction to fireworks steadily improved. While he remained attentive to the noises, his distress and efforts to conceal diminished dramatically. Rocky was able to enjoy various activities during fireworks displays, showing a good adjustment in his emotional condition.

CHAPTER 8: EXPERT INSIGHTS - VETERINARY HOMEOPATHS ON ANXIETY RELIEF IN DOGS

In this chapter, we will obtain useful insights from qualified veterinary homeopaths about the use of homeopathy for anxiety reduction in dogs. These practitioners have vast expertise in employing homeopathic principles to manage emotional imbalances and behavioral disorders in dogs. Their insights offer light on the usefulness of homeopathy and its combination with conventional veterinarian treatment in improving the emotional well-being of our beloved pets.

8.1 Interview With Dr. Emily Rodriguez, BVMS, MRCVS, VetMFHom

Q: How does homeopathy differ from conventional therapy in handling anxiety in dogs?

Dr. Rodriguez: Homeopathy offers a comprehensive approach, including the emotional, mental, and physical components of the dog. It tries to treat the fundamental cause of anxiety rather than merely suppressing symptoms. Unlike certain conventional therapies that may have side effects or brief relief, homeopathy strives to give gentle and enduring healing without causing damage.

Q: How might homeopathy support behavioral training in anxiety management?

Dr. Rodriguez: Homeopathy may considerably boost the efficiency of behavioral training. By supporting the dog's emotional well-being, homeopathy helps generate a more responsive and resilient condition, improving the learning process. Additionally, homeopathic treatments may assist in lowering anxiety, making it simpler for dogs to deal with behavioral training approaches and acquire new, calmer habits.

8.2 Interview With Dr. Mark Williams, DVM, CVA, CVCH

Q: How do you approach individualizing homeopathic treatments for dogs with anxiety?

Dr. Williams: Individualization is at the basis of homeopathy. When treating dogs with anxiety, I carefully monitor the dog's behavior, behaviors, and particular triggers. I take into mind their particular personality and temperament. By comparing these traits to the symptom picture of homeopathic medicine, I may determine the best-suited therapy for each dog's emotional requirements.

Q: What have been any noteworthy results with homeopathy for anxiety alleviation in dogs?

Dr. Williams: I've noticed great results in dogs with varied anxiety triggers. For instance, a Labrador with storm anxiety exhibited tremendous improvement with Gelsemium. A rescue dog with significant separation anxiety reacted favorably to the Arsenicum album. The personalized technique of homeopathy helps us to treat certain fears efficiently.

8.3 Interview With Dr. Jessica Lee, DVM, CCH

Q: How may pet owners incorporate homeopathy with standard veterinarian therapy for anxiety management?

Dr. Lee: Integrating homeopathy with standard veterinary treatment includes cooperation between veterinary experts and licensed veterinary homeopaths. Together, we build complete treatment regimens that incorporate both physical health and mental well-being. By combining conventional therapies with tailored homeopathic medicines, we can enhance anxiety reduction for pets.

Q: What recommendations would you provide to pet owners contemplating homeopathy for their dog's anxiety?

Dr. Lee: I would recommend pet owners seek help from a professional veterinary homeopath who can properly analyze their dog's symptoms and mental condition. Homeopathy is a mild and safe treatment, but it takes competence to identify the best suitable remedy. By engaging with a skilled specialist, pet owners may assure the greatest possible conclusion for their dog's anxiety alleviation journey.

CHAPTER 9: NUTRITIONAL SUPPORT FOR ANXIOUS DOGS

In this chapter, we will discuss the role of dietary assistance in controlling anxiety in dogs. Just like humans, a balanced and suitable diet plays a significant part in supporting emotional well-being and general health in our canine friends. By knowing the important nutrients and dietary factors, we can give tailored nutritional assistance to help decrease anxiety and foster a calmer, more balanced temperament in nervous dogs.

9.1 Essential Nutrients For Anxiety Relief

Certain nutrients have been related to lowering anxiety and fostering calm in dogs. Including these critical nutrients in a dog's diet may contribute to their mental well-being and help manage anxiety more successfully.

1. Omega-3 Fatty Acids: Omega-3 fatty acids, such as EPA and DHA, have anti-inflammatory characteristics and are proven to improve brain function. These fatty acids may help alleviate anxiety and promote cognitive function in dogs.

2. B Vitamins: B vitamins, notably B6 and B12, play a critical role in the creation of neurotransmitters in the brain, including serotonin and dopamine. These neurotransmitters are critical for controlling mood and emotions, making B vitamins essential for anxiety reduction.

3. Magnesium: Magnesium is a mineral that has soothing effects on the neurological system. It may help relieve stress and anxiety in dogs by increasing relaxation and lowering muscular tension.

4. L-Theanine: L-Theanine is an amino acid present in green tea that has soothing qualities. It may help relieve anxiety and produce a feeling of tranquility in dogs.

9.2 Foods Rich In Anxiety-reducing Nutrients

To give nutritional assistance to nervous dogs, try introducing the following items into their diet:

- Fatty Fish (e.g., salmon, mackerel, sardines) for Omega-3 fatty acids
- Lean Meat (e.g., chicken, turkey) for B vitamins
- Pumpkin Seeds and Spinach for Magnesium
- Green Tea Extract for L-Theanine

9.3 Avoiding Triggers And Allergens

In addition to adding anxiety-reducing nutrients, it is crucial to avoid specific dietary triggers and allergens that may worsen anxiety in dogs. Some dogs may be sensitive to particular substances, such as grains or certain proteins, leading to increased anxiety or restlessness. Identifying and removing these triggers from their diet might assist in a calmer temperament.

9.4 Consultation With A Veterinary Nutritionist

For dogs with severe anxiety or complicated nutritional demands, seeing a veterinarian nutritionist is suggested. A veterinary nutritionist may build a customized meal plan that meets the dog's individual anxiety triggers and nutritional needs.

CHAPTER 10: MINDFULNESS AND RELAXATION TECHNIQUES FOR DOGS

In this chapter, we will investigate the advantages of mindfulness and relaxation practices for dogs in reducing anxiety and boosting emotional well-being. Mindfulness, a condition of present-moment awareness, and relaxation activities may help dogs manage stress, decrease anxiety, and produce a feeling of tranquility. By adding these practices into their daily routine, we may help our canine friends in having a more balanced and emotionally healthy existence.

10.1 Mindfulness For Dogs

Mindfulness entails being present in the now, without judgment or attachment to past or future ideas. While dogs may not comprehend the notion of mindfulness like people do, they naturally exemplify mindfulness in their behavior. Observing and learning from our dogs' intrinsic awareness may help improve our relationship with them and provide a feeling of peace for both parties.

1 Mindful Walks

During walks with your dog, practice mindful walking by being completely present with each step. Observe your dog's behavior and responses to the surroundings. Pay attention to their body language, tail wagging, and sniffing. Engaging in mindful walks helps you to enjoy the basic delights of spending time with your dog and deepens your relationship.

2 Mindful Playtime

During playing, concentrate entirely on engaging with your dog. Remove distractions such as phones or computers. Engage in interactive games or toy play, and be attentive to your dog's answers and satisfaction. Mindful playfulness boosts the quality of your relationship, increasing your dog's emotional experience.

10.2 Relaxation Techniques For Dogs

Relaxation exercises may help dogs relieve stress, decrease anxiety, and foster a feeling of peace. Incorporating these activities into daily routines helps create a tranquil and pleasant atmosphere.

1 Breathing Exercises

Similar to people, dogs may benefit from breathing exercises. Encourage your dog to take deep breaths by utilizing slow and steady breathing. Place your hand on their chest to feel the rhythm of their breathing. This method may assist relax their nervous system and lessen anxiety.

2 Massage and TTouch

Gentle massage and TTouch (Tellington Touch) methods may improve calm in dogs. Use gentle and rhythmic strokes on their back, neck, and shoulders. TTouch utilizes circular motions on particular parts of the body to provide a relaxing effect. These methods may relieve muscular tension and help your dog relax.

3 Calming Music or White Noise

Playing gentle, tranquil music or white noise in the background might create a pleasant ambiance for your dog. This may be especially beneficial during thunderstorms, fireworks, or other anxiety-inducing events.

10.3 Creating A Safe Space

Designate a special spot in your house as a safe zone for your dog to retire to when they feel frightened or overwhelmed. Make this place cozy and appealing, with their favorite toys, bedding, and familiar odors. Encourage children to utilize this location during times of stress to help them feel safe.

CHAPTER 11: CALMING ENVIRONMENTS: CREATING A SAFE HAVEN FOR DOGS

This chapter addresses the benefits of establishing a relaxing atmosphere for dogs to help decrease anxiety and improve mental well-being. Dogs, like people, thrive in situations that give a feeling of safety, comfort, and regularity. By learning how to establish a relaxing atmosphere, we may assist our canine friends to feel more comfortable and relaxed, adding to their general happiness and pleasure.

11.1 Minimizing Noise Pollution

Noise pollution may be a major cause of worry for dogs. Loud sounds, such as fireworks, thunderstorms, or even home appliances, may provoke anxiety and stress reactions. To create a relaxing setting, consider the following:

1. *Soundproofing:* Use soundproofing materials in your house to lessen exterior noise. This might involve weather stripping on doors and windows and utilizing rugs or drapes to muffle the sound.

2. *White Noise:* Providing relaxing white noise, such as a low-volume fan or a white noise generator, may help disguise abrupt disturbances and provide a pleasant background environment.

11.2 Creating a Safe and Cozy Den

Dogs want refuge and protection, particularly during times of stress. Designate a distinct location in your house as your dog's den or safe spot. Consider the following while building up this area:

1. *Comfy Bedding:* Provide a nice and comfy bed or blanket for your dog to lay on. Having their aroma on the mattress may also bring confidence.

2. *Low Lighting:* Keep the den space gently lit with low lighting. This may generate a tranquil and secure environment.

3. *Relaxing smells:* Using aromatherapy with relaxing smells like lavender or chamomile might help relieve your dog's anxiety.

11.3 Predictable Daily Routine

Dogs thrive on regularity and consistency. A predictable daily routine may create a feeling of security and stability. Aim to create regular periods for eating, playing, walking, and relaxation. Predictable routines may help alleviate anxiety by limiting unpredictability.

11.4 Interaction and Bonding Time

Spending quality time with your dog is vital for their mental well-being. Engage in interactive play, grooming, and bonding activities to build your relationship. The time spent together may build a feeling of trust and security, lowering anxiety in your dog.

11.5 Gentle Music or TV

Leaving on quiet, mellow music or playing relaxing natural sounds while you are not at home might help create a tranquil environment for your dog. The background noise may assist disguise abrupt disturbances from the outside and lessen tension.

CHAPTER 12: HERBAL REMEDIES FOR CANINE ANXIETY

In this chapter, we will study the use of herbal treatments as a natural and holistic approach to addressing canine anxiety. Herbal medicines have been used for millennia to induce relaxation, relieve stress, and improve mental well-being in both people and animals. When provided carefully and under the advice of a veterinary practitioner, herbal therapies may offer gentle and effective assistance for nervous dogs without the possible side effects of prescription drugs.

12.1 Chamomile (Matricaria Chamomilla)

Chamomile is a well-known herbal medicine with relaxing qualities. It includes chemicals like chamazulene and apigenin, which have relaxing effects on the neurological system. Chamomile may be supplied as tea, added to the dog's diet, or used in aromatherapy to create a relaxing atmosphere.

12.2 Valerian (Valeriana officinalis)

Valerian is a natural sedative that may help decrease anxiety and promote calm in dogs. It works by boosting the amounts of gamma-aminobutyric acid (GABA) in the brain, which has a calming effect. Valerian is accessible in numerous forms, including capsules, liquid extracts, and teas.

12.3 Lemon Balm (Melissa officinalis)

Lemon balm is a soothing plant that might help reduce anxiety and uneasiness in dogs. It includes chemicals including rosmarinic acid and flavonoids, which have soothing qualities. Lemon balm may be offered as a tea or in tincture form.

12.4 Passionflower (Passiflora Incarnata)

Passionflower is recognized for its tranquilizing and calming properties. It helps decrease restlessness and anxiousness in dogs by raising GABA levels in the brain. Passionflower is accessible in many forms, including capsules, liquid extracts, and teas.

12.5 Ashwagandha (Withania somnifera)

Ashwagandha is an adaptogenic herb that may help dogs deal with stress and anxiety. It works by regulating the adrenal glands and aiding the body's stress response. Ashwagandha is available in powdered form or as a supplement.

12.6 Skullcap (Scutellaria Lateriflora)

Skullcap is a relaxing herb that might be good for dogs with anxiety and anxiousness. It includes flavonoids that have a soothing effect on the central nervous system. Skullcap is available in tincture form or as a supplement.

12.7 Using Herbal Remedies Safely

Before providing any herbal cure to your dog, it is vital to speak with a competent veterinary practitioner, such as a veterinary herbalist or holistic veterinarian. They can analyze your dog's particular requirements, health condition, and any possible interactions with drugs. Dosage and administration recommendations should be followed carefully to guarantee the safety and efficacy of the herbal treatment.

CHAPTER 13: DEALING WITH SEPARATION ANXIETY

Separation anxiety is a frequent behavioral problem in dogs and develops when they get frightened and nervous when left alone. It may lead to destructive behaviors, excessive barking, and even self-harm. In this chapter, we will examine ideas and approaches to assist dogs to manage separation anxiety, promoting a feeling of security and comfort when their owners are not there.

13.1 Gradual Desensitization

Gradual desensitization is a training strategy that helps dogs feel more comfortable with being alone. Start by leaving your dog alone for small durations, just a few minutes at a time, and gradually extend the length as your dog gets more comfortable. Pair this teaching with positive reinforcement, like sweets or toys, to build a good relationship with alone time.

13.2 Create A Safe Space

Designate a distinct location in your house as your dog's safe spot or den. Make it comfy and appealing with their favorite toys, bedding, and familiar odors. Associating this location with happy events might help your dog feel more safe when left alone.

13.3 Establish A Predictable Routine

Dogs thrive on regularity and consistency. Set a daily plan for feeding, walking, playing, and relaxation. Having a steady schedule might help alleviate anxiety by eliminating ambiguity.

13.4 Departure And Return Calmness

When leaving and coming home, have a calm manner. Avoid making a huge deal during departures and arrivals, since this might increase your dog's nervousness. Instead, keep welcomes low-key to educate your dog that absences and returns are usual and nothing to be worried about.

13.5 Interactive Toys And Puzzles

Provide your dog with engaging toys and puzzles to keep them cognitively busy during alone time. These toys may be packed with rewards or food, encouraging your dog to interact with them and diverting them from any worried sensations.

13.6 Implementing Music Or White Noise

Playing relaxing music or white noise in the background may help block out extraneous noises and create a pleasant mood. This may be especially useful for dogs with noise sensitivity or those that feel worried due to external disruptions.

13.7 Seek Professional Support

If your dog's separation anxiety is severe or does not improve with these measures, consider getting expert treatment. A trained veterinarian behaviorist or a skilled dog trainer versed in separation anxiety may give individualized instruction and training approaches to meet your dog's unique requirements.

CHAPTER 14: CANINE COMMUNICATION: UNDERSTANDING AND RESPONDING TO DOGS' SIGNALS

Effective communication is vital in creating a deep and trustworthy relationship with our canine friends. Dogs have their particular methods of expressing themselves via body language, vocalizations, and actions. In this chapter, we will study the numerous signs that dogs use to communicate and how humans might better comprehend and react to their cues, establishing a stronger relationship and mutual understanding.

14.1 Body Language

Dogs largely communicate via body language. Understanding their postures and motions might reveal vital insights into their emotional state and goals.

1. Tail Wagging: A wagging tail may signify many emotions. A wide and loose wag normally signifies enjoyment and friendliness, whereas a stiff and high wag may suggest attention or caution.

2. *Ears:* Erect and forward-facing ears frequently express alertness or curiosity, whereas flattened ears may imply fear or submission.

3. *Eye Contact:* Direct eye contact may express boldness or challenge, while a gentle look is a sign of trust and love.

4. *Lip Licking:* Dogs may lick their lips as a soothing indication, particularly when they feel worried or uncomfortable.

5. *Paw Lifting:* Raising a paw may be a technique for a dog to seek attention or communicate hesitation.

6. *Body Posture:* A relaxed and fluid body posture reflects a pleasant and satisfied attitude, whereas a stiff or hunched posture may indicate dread or worry.

14.2 Vocalizations

Dogs employ diverse vocalizations to convey their wants and feelings.

1. *Barking:* Barking might signify enthusiasm, fear, awareness, or a need for attention. The pitch and intensity of the bark might reveal indications about the underlying mood.

2. *Whining:* Whining may be a method for dogs to convey worry, discomfort, or a desire for something.

3. *Howling:* Howling is typically a communication between dogs, but it may also be a reaction to specific noises or emotions of loneliness.

14.3 Responding To Dogs' Signals

To encourage successful communication with our dogs, it is necessary to react correctly to their cues.

1. *Be Attentive:* Pay great attention to your dog's body language and vocalizations. Understanding their indications helps you to react immediately to their requirements.

2. *Respect Personal Space:* Give your dog the space they need when they exhibit indications of discomfort or distress. Forcing encounters may exacerbate stress and undermine trust.

3. *good Reinforcement:* Reward good actions and responses with rewards, praise, or love. Positive reinforcement builds the link between you and your dog.

4. *Training and Socialization:* Proper training and socialization may help dogs gain confidence and improve communication abilities. Positive relationships with other dogs and humans contribute to their emotional well-being.

CHAPTER 15: FUTURE TRENDS IN HOMEOPATHIC ANXIETY RELIEF FOR DOGS

As the area of homeopathic medicine continues to improve, we may predict interesting future trends in anxiety alleviation for dogs. Homeopathy provides a natural and holistic approach to fostering emotional well-being in our canine friends. In this chapter, we will examine some possible future possibilities and developments in homeopathic anxiety reduction for dogs, anticipating a better and more compassionate future for their care.

15.1 Advanced Research And Evidence-Based Practice

The future of homeopathic anxiety therapy for dogs will likely witness an increase in scientific study and evidence-based practice. As more researchers concentrate on examining the efficacy of homeopathic treatments, we should anticipate an increasing body of data supporting their use in controlling canine anxiety. This study will give significant insights into the exact medicines and regimens that work best for various forms of anxiety in dogs.

15.2 Personalized Treatment Plans

Advancements in technology and customized medicine will allow the construction of individualized treatment strategies for dogs with anxiety. By evaluating a dog's distinctive health history, genetics, and behavioral patterns, veterinary homeopaths may produce exact medicines that address their unique anxiety triggers and demands. Personalized therapy strategies will lead to more effective and tailored relief for stressed pets.

15.3 Integration With Behavioral Therapy

The future will certainly bring further integration of homeopathic anxiety alleviation with behavioral treatment. Combining homeopathic medications with behavioral approaches may give a holistic approach to controlling anxiety in dogs. Behavioral therapy may assist alter bad habits and teach coping methods, while homeopathy encourages emotional balance and well-being.

15.4 Telehealth Consultations

Advancements in telehealth technology will allow pet owners to obtain homeopathic consultations from the comfort of their homes. Virtual consultations with trained veterinary homeopaths will become more available, making it simpler for pet owners to obtain professional advice and assistance for their worried pets.

15.5 Herbal And Nutraceutical Combinations

In the future, homeopathic medicines may be paired with herbal supplements and nutraceuticals to boost anxiety reduction. The synergistic impact of these natural therapies may give a complete and well-rounded therapy for dogs with anxiety.

15.6 Stress-Reducing Environments

As our awareness of the influence of the environment on canine anxiety develops, future trends may concentrate on establishing stress-reducing surroundings for dogs. Integrating homeopathy with environmental adjustments, such as calming aromas, soothing music, and designated safe places, may contribute to a more relaxing and anxiety-free situation for our animal companions.

CONCLUSION

In this thorough book, we have dived into the area of homeopathic anxiety medication for dogs, covering all facets of this holistic approach to improving the mental well-being of our canine friends. From learning the historical backdrop and essential ideas of homeopathy to researching its practical uses and future trends, we have learned vital insights into how this gentle and compassionate type of therapy may positively benefit our animal pets.

Throughout the chapters, we have learned about the need for a well-structured and tailored approach to anxiety reduction for dogs. By knowing the individual requirements and triggers of each dog, we can create remedies and treatment programs to give the most effective and focused care. From behavioral training and mindfulness methods to dietary assistance and herbal medicines, the combination of numerous holistic therapies increases the entire well-being of our canine friends.

As someone with competence in veterinary medicine and more than a decade of experience, I hope this book serves as a beneficial resource for anyone interested in getting a comprehensive grasp of homeopathic anxiety therapy for dogs. By addressing frequent difficulties, presenting real-life examples, and investigating future trends, this book seeks to empower pet owners and veterinary professionals with the information and resources to effectively help nervous dogs in their care.

It is crucial to underline the relevance of getting expert assistance and consultation from licensed veterinary homeopaths or holistic veterinarians before beginning a homeopathic treatment journey for dogs with anxiety. Their skill and experience can assure the safe and successful administration of homeopathic medications, and provide specialized treatment suited to each dog's particular requirements.

In conclusion, the well-being of our furry pets is of the highest significance. By cultivating a greater awareness of homeopathy and its role in anxiety alleviation, we may establish a more compassionate and holistic approach to caring for our beloved pets. With commitment, patience, and love, we can help our canine friends experience happier, healthier, and anxiety-free lives, deepening the link between people and dogs for years to come.

Bonus

POSITIVE REINFORCEMENT TRAINING MASTERCLASS FOR DOGS

Introducing the Positive Reinforcement Training Masterclass for Dogs

Are you ready to embark on a journey of joyful learning and bonding with your furry companion? Welcome to the Positive Reinforcement Training Masterclass for Dogs, a transformative experience designed to enhance your relationship with your canine friend through the power of positive reinforcement.

Why Positive Reinforcement Training?

Positive reinforcement training is a force-free and compassionate approach to teaching your dog new behaviors and strengthening their existing skills. It focuses on rewarding desired behaviors with treats, praise, and play, creating a fun and engaging learning environment for your dog. By celebrating their successes, you build trust and deepen the bond with your furry companion.

Who is this Masterclass For?

Whether you have a new puppy eager to learn or an older dog seeking to brush up on their skills, this masterclass is for every dog owner who believes in nurturing a harmonious and loving relationship with their pet. No prior training experience is necessary; all you need is a willingness to learn and a heart full of love for your canine companion.

What Will You Learn?

In this masterclass, you will gain a comprehensive understanding of positive reinforcement training techniques and principles. From basic commands like "sit" and "stay" to more advanced tricks, you'll discover how to effectively communicate with your dog and build a foundation for a lifetime of learning and growth.

You'll explore ways to capture your dog's attention and maintain focus, even in distracting situations. Our expert trainers will guide you through hands-on exercises that foster engagement and create positive associations with training.

The Transformative Power of Positive Reinforcement

At the heart of this masterclass lies the transformative power of positive reinforcement. You'll witness how gentle encouragement and rewards can shape your dog's behavior and encourage a desire to please. This creates a positive training experience that not only brings joy to your furry friend but also strengthens your connection as a team.

Our Commitment to Force-Free Training

In this masterclass, you can rest assured that we promote only force-free and kind training methods. We believe that building trust and fostering a positive bond are essential for a happy and well-adjusted dog. You'll learn how to address behavior challenges with patience and compassion, empowering your dog to thrive in a supportive environment.

Join Us on this Journey of Love and Learning

We invite you to join us on this journey of love and learning with your furry companion. Our Positive Reinforcement Training Masterclass for Dogs is an opportunity to discover the joy of training and witness the incredible transformations that positive reinforcement can bring to your dog's behavior and emotional well-being.

Enroll now and unlock the potential of positive reinforcement training in your dog's life. Wagging tails, happy barks, and a world of shared adventures await as you embark on this enriching journey together. Let's create a positive and loving training experience for your dog, and let the learning and bonding begin!

MODULE 1: UNDERSTANDING POSITIVE REINFORCEMENT TRAINING

Positive reinforcement training is a compassionate and effective approach to teaching and guiding dogs, based on the principle of rewarding desired behaviors to encourage their repetition. This foundational module of the Positive Reinforcement Training Masterclass for Dogs lays the groundwork for a successful and fulfilling training journey, fostering a strong bond between you and your furry companion.

The Power of Positive Reinforcement

At the heart of positive reinforcement training lies the power of rewards. By offering treats, praise, or play as rewards for desired behaviors, we create positive associations, making your dog more likely to offer those behaviors willingly. This approach focuses on building motivation and cooperation rather than using force or punishment. The result is a happy and confident dog who is eager to learn and please.

Positive reinforcement goes beyond shaping behaviors; it nurtures a trusting and respectful relationship between you and your dog. By focusing on the positive, we create a harmonious training environment that fosters emotional well-being and a strong sense of trust.

The Science Of Positive Reinforcement

Positive reinforcement training is not just a feel-good approach; it is deeply rooted in scientific principles. Understanding the science behind it enhances our appreciation for its effectiveness.

Operant conditioning is a fundamental concept in positive reinforcement training. It involves associating specific actions with consequences. When a behavior is followed by a reward, the likelihood of that behavior being repeated increases. Over time, this process strengthens the connection between the behavior and the reward.

Positive reinforcement also triggers the release of neurotransmitters like dopamine in the brain, creating a positive feedback loop. This reinforces the connection between the behavior and the rewarding experience, making your dog more motivated to perform the desired action.

Clear Communication And Timing

For positive reinforcement to be effective, clear communication and impeccable timing are essential. Your dog needs to understand which behaviors are being rewarded, so timely and precise delivery of rewards is crucial.

Use verbal cues, such as "good" or "yes," to mark the desired behavior the moment it happens. This is known as a "marker" and acts as a bridge between the behavior and the reward, allowing your dog to associate the two.

Rewarding your dog within a few seconds of the desired behavior reinforces the connection, making it easier for your dog to understand what you are asking of them. Be consistent in your communication and timing to avoid confusion and maintain clarity during training.

Building A Positive Training Environment

Creating a positive training environment sets the stage for successful learning experiences. Choose a quiet and distraction-free space where your dog can focus on the training. Keep training sessions short and enjoyable, and end on a positive note to leave your dog eager for the next session.

Set realistic goals for each training session, breaking complex behaviors into smaller, achievable steps. This prevents your dog from becoming overwhelmed and allows for incremental progress.

Adapt your training approach to suit your dog's individual needs and personality. Some dogs may be highly motivated by treats, while others may prefer praise or play. Understanding what motivates your dog best helps tailor the training experience to their preferences.

Building Trust and Strengthening the Bond

Positive reinforcement training is an opportunity to strengthen the bond between you and your dog. Focus on nurturing a trusting relationship through kindness, patience, and empathy.

Be a patient and supportive teacher, avoiding frustration or impatience during training. Celebrate even the smallest successes, and offer encouragement and affection to build your dog's confidence.

Empower your dog to make choices during training, allowing them to offer behaviors and engage in problem-solving. This sense of agency fosters a sense of partnership and mutual understanding.

Above all, training sessions should be enjoyable and stress-free for both you and your dog. Embrace a positive and lighthearted attitude, and watch as your dog becomes an eager and willing learner.

Embracing Mistakes As Learning Opportunities

In the process of training, mistakes are inevitable and should be embraced as learning opportunities. Instead of becoming discouraged, view mistakes as valuable feedback to guide your training approach.

If your dog doesn't respond as expected, consider adjusting your communication, timing, or training technique. Be patient and flexible in your approach, allowing room for trial and error.

Avoid punishment or scolding, as this can create fear and anxiety, hindering the learning process. Instead, redirect your dog's behavior towards the desired action and reinforce it positively.

MODULE 2: BUILDING FOCUS AND ENGAGEMENT

Welcome to Module 2 of the Positive Reinforcement Training Masterclass for Dogs! In this module, we'll explore techniques to capture your dog's focus and maintain their engagement during training sessions. Building focus and engagement are crucial for successful learning experiences, creating a strong connection between you and your furry companion.

The Importance Of Focus And Engagement

Focus and engagement are the cornerstones of effective training. When your dog is focused on you, they are more receptive to learning and following your cues. Engaging your dog in the training process not only enhances their motivation but also strengthens the bond between you.

A focused and engaged dog is more likely to offer desired behaviors willingly, making the training experience enjoyable and rewarding for both of you. By nurturing focus and engagement, you lay the foundation for a positive and productive training journey.

Capturing Your Dog's Attention

Capturing your dog's attention is the first step toward building focus. In this section, we'll explore techniques to redirect your dog's focus toward you during training sessions.

Use a verbal cue, such as their name, to get your dog's attention. When they look at you, immediately mark the behavior with a "good" or "yes" and offer a reward. Practice this exercise in a quiet and distraction-free environment, gradually increasing the level of distractions as your dog becomes more proficient.

Avoid using force or harsh commands to get your dog's attention, as this can create anxiety and hinder focus. Instead, be patient and gentle in redirecting their attention towards you.

Maintaining Engagement Through Play

Play is a powerful tool for maintaining your dog's engagement during training. Incorporating play into training sessions not only adds an element of fun but also reinforces the connection between you and your dog.

Use interactive toys, such as tug ropes or fetch balls, to initiate play sessions. Engage in short bursts of play between training exercises to keep your dog's enthusiasm high. Remember to use play as a reward for a job well done during training, creating positive associations with learning.

Observe your dog's body language during play to ensure they are enjoying the interaction. Tail wags, play bows, and eager expressions are signs of a happy and engaged dog.

Building Focus In Challenging Environments

Training in challenging environments is essential for real-life applications. In this section, we'll discuss techniques to build focus in distracting settings.

Start training in a low-distraction environment and gradually add distractions as your dog becomes more proficient. Use high-value rewards, such as extra tasty treats or favorite toys, to maintain their focus in challenging situations.

Practice "leave it" exercises to teach your dog to ignore distractions and maintain focus on you. Reward them generously when they respond appropriately to distractions, reinforcing the desired behavior.

Be patient and understanding during this process, as building focus in challenging environments takes time and practice. Celebrate small victories and progress, and avoid overwhelming your dog with too many distractions at once.

Games For Focus And Engagement

Games are an enjoyable way to enhance focus and engagement. In this section, we'll introduce interactive games that promote mental stimulation and build your dog's focus.

Find It: Hide treats or toys around the room and encourage your dog to search for them using their nose. This game not only sharpens their scenting skills but also keeps them engaged and mentally stimulated.

Touch: Teach your dog to touch its nose to your hand or a target object. This game builds focus and strengthens your communication with your dog.

Name Game: Encourage your dog to respond to their name by offering rewards when they look at you upon hearing their name. This reinforces their name as a cue for attention and focus.

MODULE 3: BASIC COMMANDS AND MANNERS

Welcome to Module 3 of the Positive Reinforcement Training Masterclass for Dogs! In this module, we'll delve into teaching your furry companion essential basic commands and good manners. These fundamental skills are the building blocks of a well-behaved, obedient dog, and also form the foundation for more advanced training.

The Importance Of Basic Commands And Manners

Basic commands and manners are essential for a harmonious relationship between you and your dog. They provide clear communication and guidance, ensuring your dog understands what is expected of them in various situations.

Teaching basic commands not only enhances your dog's responsiveness but also promotes their safety and the safety of those around them. Good manners, such as polite leash walking and waiting at doors, make daily interactions enjoyable and stress-free.

Teaching "Sit"

"Sit" is one of the most fundamental commands every dog should learn. It establishes impulse control and serves as a foundation for other behaviors.

To teach "sit," hold a treat close to your dog's nose and slowly raise it above its head. As their head follows the treat, their bottom will naturally lower into a sitting position. The moment they sit, mark the behavior with a "good" or "yes" and reward them with the treat.

Practice this command in different environments and gradually phase out the use of treats, replacing them with praise and affection as rewards.

Teaching "Stay"

"Stay" is a valuable command that helps keep your dog safe and under control in various situations.

Start with your dog in a sitting or standing position. Extend your hand, palm facing your dog, and say "stay" in a calm and clear voice. Take a step back and wait for a few seconds before returning to your dog. If they stay in place, mark the behavior with a "good" or "yes" and reward them with a treat.

Gradually increase the duration and distance of the "stay" command, always returning to your dog to release them from the stay position.

Teaching "Leave It"

"Leave it" is a crucial command that prevents your dog from picking up or engaging with unwanted items or distractions.

Hold a treat in your closed hand and present it to your dog, saying "leave it" as they show interest. When your dog stops trying to get the treat, mark the behavior with a "good" or "yes" and offer them a different, more desirable treat from your other hand.

Practice "leave it" with various objects and distractions, reinforcing the command with rewards for appropriate responses.

Teaching Polite Leash Walking

Polite leash walking is essential for enjoyable walks and outdoor adventures with your dog.

Start by standing still whenever your dog pulls on the leash. When they return to your side, mark the behavior with a "good" or "yes" and reward them with a treat. This teaches your dog that pulling on the leash results in no progress while walking politely is rewarded.

Use the "heel" command to encourage your dog to walk calmly beside you. Hold a treat at your side and start walking, saying "heel" as your dog follows you. Reward them for staying in the proper position.

Be patient and consistent during leash walking training, and avoid jerking or yanking on the leash, as this can be aversive and counterproductive.

Teaching "Wait" at Doors

Teaching your dog to "wait" at doors is essential for safety and prevents them from bolting outside.

Start with your dog on a leash or in a controlled environment near a door. As you approach the door, say "wait" and hold your dog back gently with the leash or your body.

Open the door slightly, and if your dog remains in place, mark the behavior with a "good" or "yes" and offer them a reward. Gradually increase the duration of the "wait" before allowing your dog to pass through the door.

MODULE 4: ADDRESSING BEHAVIOR CHALLENGES

Welcome to Module 4 of the Positive Reinforcement Training Masterclass for Dogs! In this module, we'll explore how to address common behavior challenges using positive reinforcement techniques. Every dog may face certain behavior issues at some point in their lives, and understanding how to handle these challenges with kindness and patience is essential for a harmonious relationship with your furry companion.

The Power of Positive Redirection

Positive redirection is a key strategy in addressing behavior challenges. Instead of punishing undesirable behaviors, we redirect our dog's attention and offer alternative behaviors that we want to reinforce.

For example, if your dog is jumping on guests, instead of scolding them, redirect their attention to a toy or treat. When they engage with the toy or take the treat politely, reward them with praise and affection. This encourages them to offer the desired behavior instead of the undesired one.

Patience and Consistency

Addressing behavior challenges requires patience and consistency. Dogs, like humans, take time to learn and adapt to new behaviors. Be patient with your furry friend as they navigate through the learning process.

Consistency is crucial in reinforcing positive behaviors and discouraging negative ones. Set clear boundaries and expectations, and ensure that all family members and caregivers are on the same page regarding training approaches.

Counter-Conditioning And Desensitization

Counter-conditioning and desensitization are effective techniques for helping your dog overcome fears and anxieties.

If your dog is fearful of thunderstorms, for example, create a positive association by offering treats, praise, or play during storms. Gradually increase the intensity of the sound while rewarding calm and relaxed behavior.

Over time, your dog will learn that storms predict positive experiences, reducing their anxiety.

Addressing Reactivity On Leash

Leash reactivity, such as barking or lunging toward other dogs or people, can be challenging to manage. Positive reinforcement can help you address this behavior.

When your dog remains calm in the presence of triggers, mark the behavior with a "good" or "yes" and reward them with treats. This reinforces the positive association with the presence of the trigger.

To create distance from the trigger, use the "leave it" and "heel" commands to redirect your dog's focus. Reward them for walking calmly beside you when they show appropriate behavior.

Coping With Separation Anxiety

Separation anxiety is a common challenge for dogs, especially when left alone. Positive reinforcement can aid in alleviating their distress.

Practice short periods of separation and reward your dog for calm behavior during these times. Gradually increase the duration of separation, always returning to your dog with a reward when they remain calm.

Create a positive environment when leaving and returning by offering treats or toys before departure and after arriving home. This helps your dog associate your departures with positive experiences.

Addressing Jumping And Excitability

Jumping and excessive excitement can be challenging behaviors to manage, especially when greeting guests.

Teach your dog an alternative behavior, such as "sit" or "down," to replace jumping when greeting. Reward them for offering alternative behavior instead.

Ask guests to ignore your dog until they are calm and sitting. When your dog approaches guests calmly, reward them with attention and treats, reinforcing the polite greeting.

MODULE 5: ADVANCED TRAINING AND TRICKS

Welcome to Module 5 of the Positive Reinforcement Training Masterclass for Dogs! In this module, we'll delve into the world of advanced training techniques and tricks. Building on the foundation of positive reinforcement, we'll explore how to challenge and stimulate your furry companion's mind, fostering a deeper connection and creating a fun and engaging training experience.

The Benefits of Advanced Training

Advanced training goes beyond basic commands and provides mental stimulation and enrichment for your dog. Teaching new and complex behaviors keeps their mind sharp and provides an outlet for their intelligence and energy.

Engaging in advanced training with your dog strengthens the bond between you and deepens mutual trust. It also provides an opportunity for you and your dog to work together as a team, accomplishing impressive feats through positive reinforcement.

Shaping Behaviors

Shaping is a technique used to teach complex behaviors by breaking them down into manageable steps. Instead of luring or guiding your dog into a position, shaping involves rewarding incremental progress toward the final behavior.

For example, to teach a "spin" trick, reward your dog for turning its head slightly to the side. Gradually increase the criteria, rewarding for a larger turn each time until your dog completes a full spin.

Shaping allows your dog to actively participate in problem-solving, increasing their confidence and enthusiasm for learning.

Capturing Behaviors

Capturing is another technique for teaching advanced behaviors. It involves observing your dog and rewarding them when they naturally offer a desired behavior.

For example, if your dog occasionally sits with their paws crossed, capture this behavior by marking and rewarding it when it happens. With repetition, your dog will start offering the crossed-paw sit more frequently, making it easier to reinforce the behavior.

Capturing allows you to train behaviors without actively promoting your dog, making it a valuable tool for shaping advanced tricks.

Teaching Complex Tricks

In this section, we'll explore a few complex tricks you can teach your dog using positive reinforcement.

"Play Dead": To teach your dog to play dead, start with them in a lying-down position. Hold a treat close to their nose and move it towards their shoulder, encouraging them to roll onto their side. When they lie on their side, mark the behavior and reward them.

"Fetch Your Toy": Teach your dog to fetch a specific toy by using the "take it" and "drop it" commands. Start by encouraging them to pick up the toy and rewarding them for doing so. Then, teach the "drop it" command, rewarding them for releasing the toy on command.

"Back Up": Teach your dog to back up on cue by gently walking towards them. As they take a step backward, mark the behavior and reward them. Gradually increase the distance they back up before rewarding.

Proofing Behaviors

Once your dog has learned advanced tricks, it's essential to prove them in different environments and with distractions.

Practice the tricks in various locations, gradually increasing the level of distractions. Offer rewards and praise for successful performances, reinforcing the tricks in different contexts.

Proofing helps solidify your dog's understanding of the behaviors and ensures they can perform them reliably, even in challenging situations.

Embracing the Joy of Learning

Advanced training and tricks are a celebration of your dog's intelligence, agility, and willingness to learn. Embrace the joy of learning together and approach each training session with enthusiasm and positivity.

Remember that advanced training requires patience and persistence. Break down complex tricks into achievable steps, and celebrate each small success along the way.

CONCLUSION

Congratulations on completing the Positive Reinforcement Training Masterclass for Dogs! Throughout this comprehensive and informative journey, you've delved into the world of positive reinforcement training, fostering a deeper understanding of this compassionate and effective approach to teaching and guiding your furry companions.

In this masterclass, we explored the core principles of positive reinforcement, understanding the power of rewards and their impact on shaping desired behaviors. You learned how to create a positive training environment, built on clear communication, patience, and consistent reinforcement, cultivating a harmonious and trusting relationship with your dog.

From mastering basic commands and manners to addressing behavior challenges with compassion and understanding, you've gained invaluable tools to navigate the ups and downs of your dog's training journey. By embracing positive redirection, counter-conditioning, and desensitization, you've empowered your dog to overcome fears and anxieties, leading to a more confident and contented companion.

As you progressed through the masterclass, you delved into the exciting realm of advanced training and tricks, stimulating your dog's mind and building a deeper bond through shared accomplishments. Shaping behaviors, capturing moments, and proofing skills in different environments have honed your training expertise and highlighted the joy of learning together.

Throughout this masterclass, we celebrated the magic of positive reinforcement, recognizing that training is not just about teaching commands but about fostering love, trust, and mutual respect. By nurturing a positive and supportive training environment, you've set the stage for a lifetime of joyful learning experiences with your furry friend.

As you continue your training journey with your dog, remember the guiding principles of this masterclass: patience, consistency, and kindness. Embrace the power of positive reinforcement as you navigate the complexities of training and behavior challenges, knowing that you are creating a lasting impact on your dog's well-being and happiness.

Thank you for investing your time and dedication in this masterclass. Your commitment to positive reinforcement training speaks volumes about your love and care for your canine companion. We hope this masterclass has empowered you to create an enriching and rewarding life together with your furry friend, filled with shared adventures, delightful tricks, and a bond that knows no bounds.

Congratulations once again on completing the Positive Reinforcement Training Masterclass for Dogs! May your journey be filled with wagging tails, happy barks, and the joy of learning and growing together. Happy training!

Dear Readers,

Thank you from the bottom of our hearts for choosing to explore "Anxiety Relief for Dogs." Your dedication to understanding and improving the well-being of your furry companions is truly commendable.

We hope this book has provided you with valuable insights, effective strategies, and a deep understanding of how to provide relief and comfort to your anxious dogs.

May the knowledge you've gained from these pages lead to a happier, calmer, and more peaceful life for both you and your beloved canine friends.

With gratitude and warm wishes,

Dr Baron Harper Sagewood

About the Author - The Baron Harper Sagewood

Dr. Baron Harper Sagewood, a distinguished veterinarian and Ph.D. holder, is not only an expert in the field of animal care but also a passionate advocate for the well-being of our beloved pets. His profound love for animals, particularly dogs, took root at the tender age of four when he received his first German Shepherd pup, a furry companion who would forever shape his life's journey.

Growing up with his loyal German Shepherd by his side, Dr. Sagewood experienced firsthand the unconditional love, loyalty, and emotional bond that can exist between a human and their four-legged friend. This early connection sparked a deep curiosity within him to understand and enhance the lives of animals through compassionate care.

Driven by his unwavering dedication, Dr. Sagewood pursued a Ph.D. in veterinary medicine, specializing in canine wellness and behavior. His extensive research and groundbreaking contributions in the field have earned him recognition among his peers and the admiration of pet owners worldwide.

Beyond his academic accomplishments, what truly sets Dr. Sagewood apart is his profound empathy and understanding of the emotional needs of dogs. He firmly believes that a harmonious relationship between humans and dogs goes beyond physical care. It requires a holistic approach that encompasses their emotional well-being, nutrition, and the power of connection.

Dr. Sagewood's expertise, combined with his genuine compassion for animals, has guided him in developing innovative approaches to canine care. His unique insights have transformed the lives of countless pets and their owners, enabling them to forge deeper bonds and create a nurturing environment filled with love and understanding.

As an author, Dr. Sagewood weaves his extensive knowledge, personal experiences, and heartfelt passion into his writings. His ability to capture the essence of the human-dog bond, to delve into the depths of their emotions, and to offer practical guidance is truly awe-inspiring. Dr. Sagewood's words have the power to uplift, inspire, and ignite a deep sense of love and devotion towards our furry companions.

Whether it's his groundbreaking research on canine nutrition, his insights into behavioral training, or his heartfelt stories of resilience and healing, Dr. Sagewood's writing resonates with pet owners around the world. His captivating storytelling, coupled with his profound understanding of the canine psyche, provides a roadmap for creating a harmonious and fulfilling life for dogs and their human companions.

Dr. Baron Harper Sagewood's lifelong commitment to the well-being of animals, his extensive knowledge, and his unwavering love for dogs make him an exceptional authority in the field of veterinary medicine. His work continues to inspire, educate, and empower pet owners to provide the best care for their beloved canine friends.

Other Books By Dr Baron Harper Sagewood

Canine Wellness
Wholesome Paws Cookbook
Healthy Homemade dog food